What's the Issue?

WHAT'S MENTAL HEALTH?

By Jennifer Lombardo

KidHaven PUBLISHING

Published in 2022 by
KidHaven Publishing, an Imprint of Greenhaven Publishing, LLC
353 3rd Avenue
Suite 255
New York, NY 10010

Designer: Deanna Paternostro
Editor: Jennifer Lombardo

Photo credits: Cover (top) Syda Productions/Shutterstock.com; cover (bottom) SewCream/Shutterstock.com; pp. 5 (top), 11 Africa Studio/Shutterstock.com; p. 5 (bottom) Kiian Oksana/Shutterstock.com; p. 7 (main) Dragon Images/Shutterstock.com; p. 7 (inset) SpeedKingz/Shutterstock.com; p. 9 (main) Eva Foreman/Shutterstock.com; p. 9 (inset) fizkes/Shutterstock.com; p. 13 pixelheadphoto digitalskillet/Shutterstock.com; p. 15 Kamira/Shutterstock.com; p. 17 (top) VGstockstudio/Shutterstock.com; p. 17 (bottom) Monkey Business Images/Shutterstock.com; pp. 19, 21 Alex Gontar/Shutterstock.com.

Library of Congress Cataloging-in-Publication Data

Names: Lombardo, Jennifer, author.
Title: What's mental health? / Jennifer Lombardo.
Description: First edition. | New York : KidHaven Publishing, [2022] | Series: What's the issue? | Includes bibliographical references and index.
Identifiers: LCCN 2019059385 (print) | LCCN 2019059386 (ebook) | ISBN 9781534534506 (library binding) | ISBN 9781534534483 (paperback) | ISBN 9781534534490 (set) | ISBN 9781534534513 (ebook)
Subjects: LCSH: Mental health–Juvenile literature. | Mental illness–Juvenile literature.
Classification: LCC RA790 .L686 2022 (print) | LCC RA790 (ebook) | DDC 616.89–dc23
LC record available at https://lccn.loc.gov/2019059385
LC ebook record available at https://lccn.loc.gov/2019059386

Printed in the United States of America

Some of the images in this book illustrate individuals who are models. The depictions do not imply actual situations or events.

CPSIA compliance information: Batch #CS22KH: For further information contact Greenhaven Publishing LLC, New York, New York at 1-844-317-7404.

Please visit our website, www.greenhavenpublishing.com. For a free color catalog of all our high-quality books, call toll free 1-844-317-7404 or fax 1-844-317-7405.

Find us on

CONTENTS

Taking Care of Yourself

You probably know that to keep your body healthy, you need to exercise and eat good foods. However, a lot of people don't know that mental health is just as important as **physical** health. Your mental health includes your mind, your feelings, and how you deal with your friends and family.

Mental health is very important because it **affects** how we think, feel, and act. Everyone needs to take care of their mental health, no matter how young or old they are. This starts with understanding what mental health is and being able to spot signs of problems with your mental health.

Facing the Facts

Some people think kids can't have mental health problems, but this isn't true. In 2013, **experts** found that kids as young as three can show symptoms, or signs, of mental **disorders**.

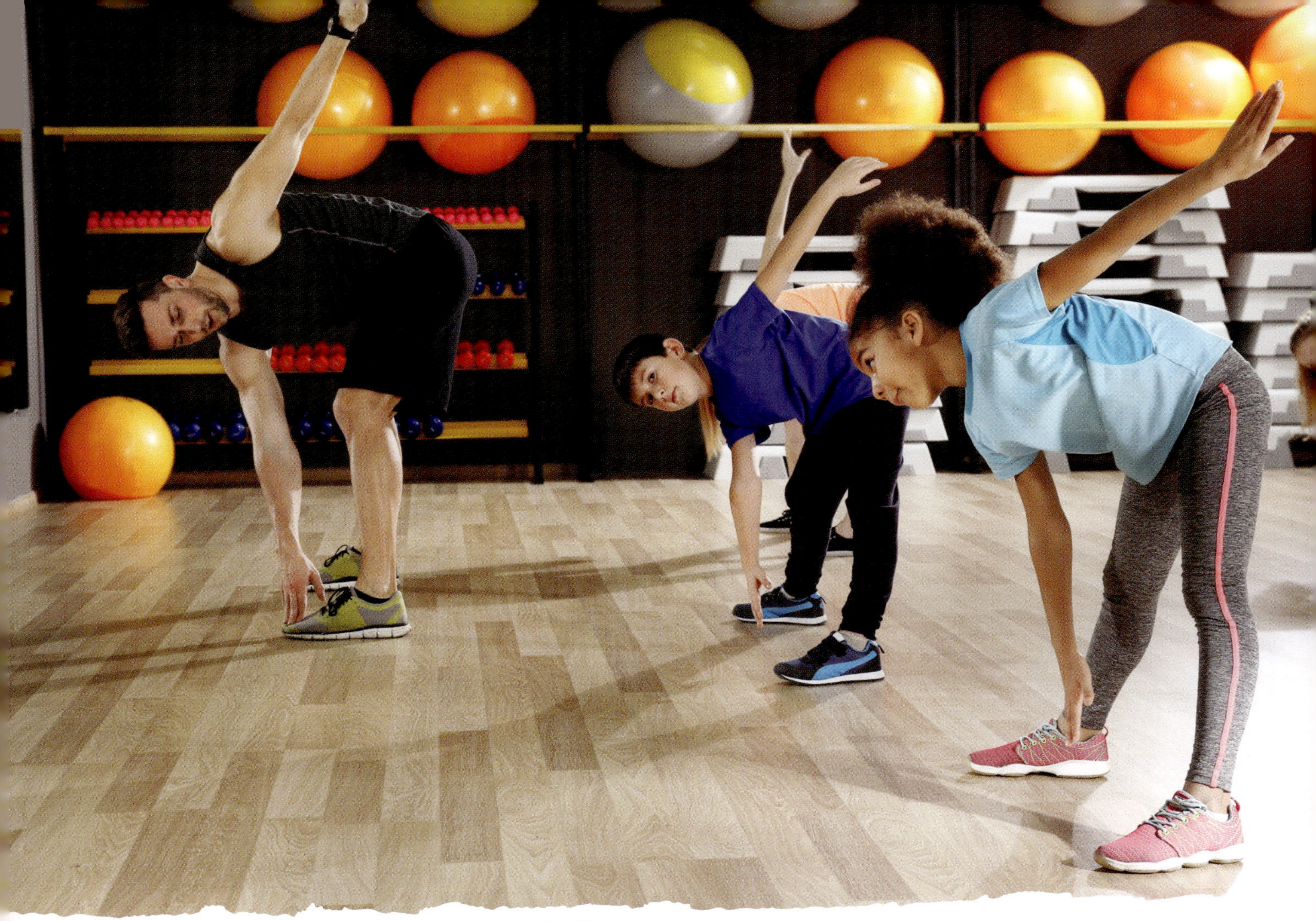

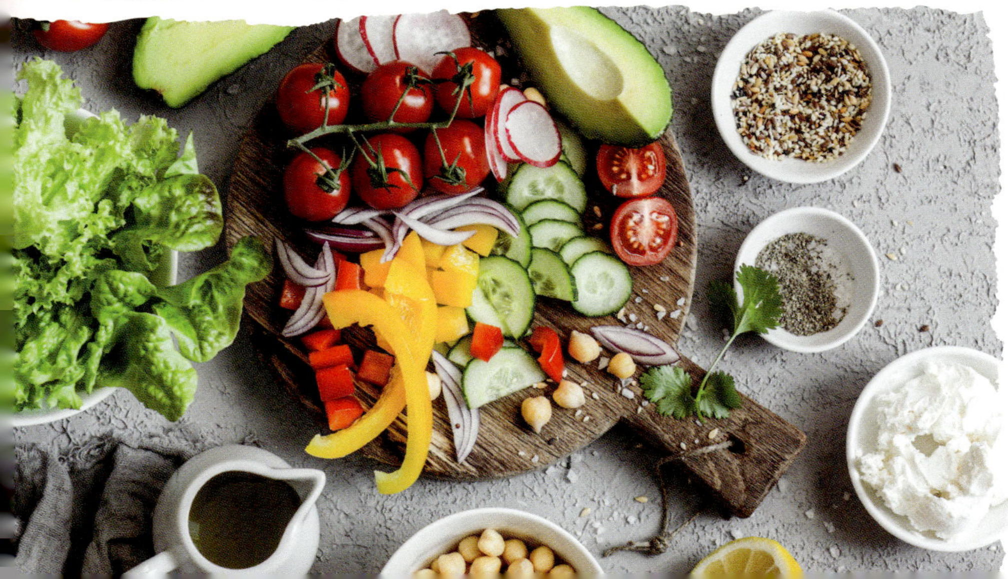

Physical and mental health are connected. When your body feels good because you're exercising and eating well, you're more likely to be in a good mood.

Dealing with Stress

Stress doesn't feel good, but it's a part of life that everyone deals with. Dealing with something unpleasant is called coping. Different people have different ways of coping. These ways of coping are called coping mechanisms.

There are good coping mechanisms and bad, or poor, coping mechanisms. People who never learn good coping mechanisms have much worse mental health. This is because poor coping mechanisms don't fix anything. In fact, they can make your problems worse. Learning what helps you cope with stress in a healthy way is an important part of having good mental health.

Facing the Facts

Stress harms your body if it goes on for too long. Some of the physical problems stress can cause are stomachaches, headaches, problems with sleeping, and sore muscles.

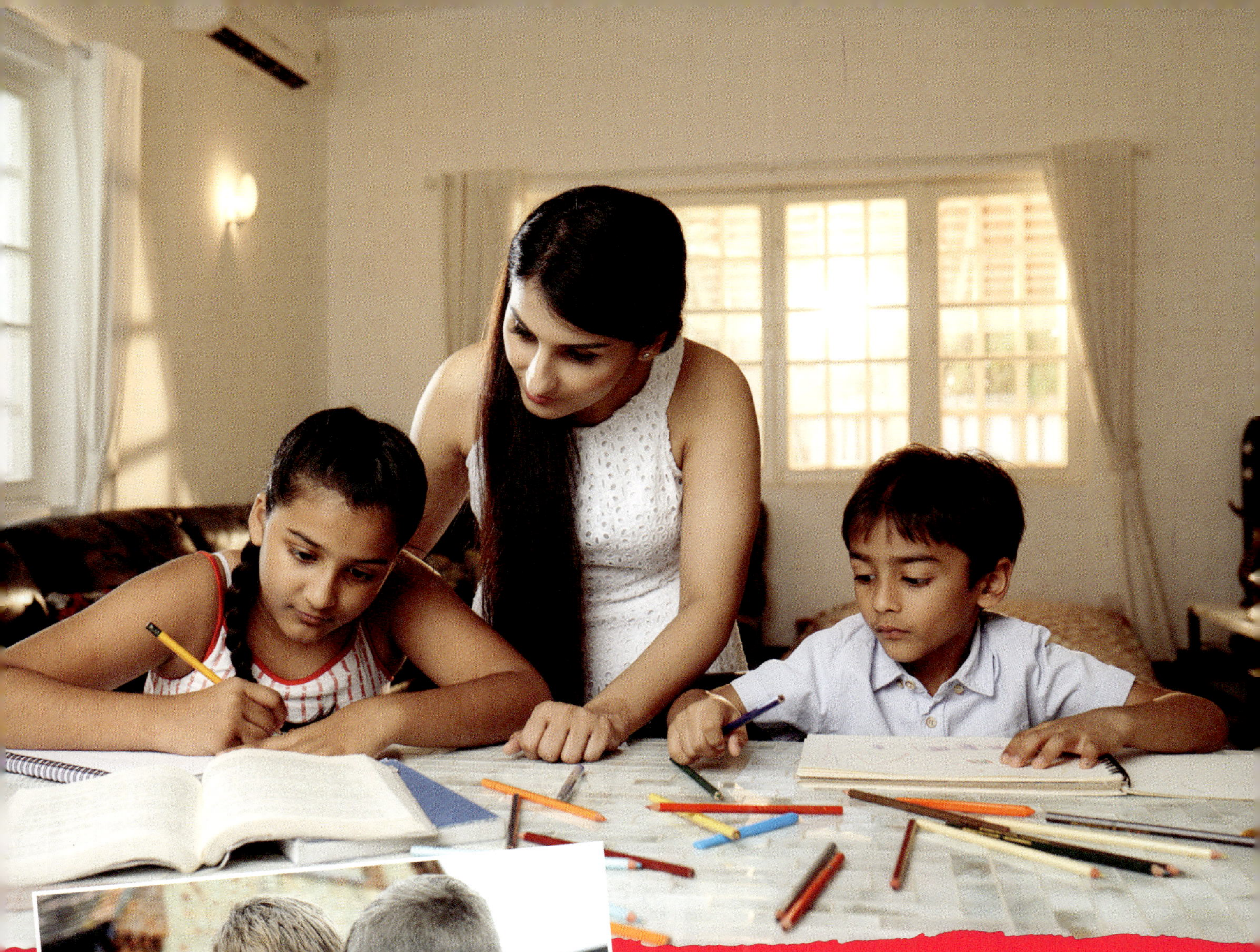

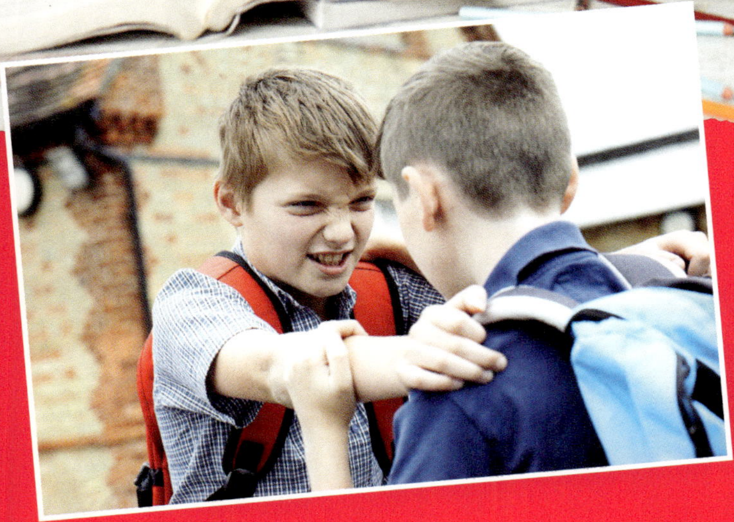

Everyone gets stressed sometimes. Things such as having a lot of homework, starting at a new school, or having a fight with a friend are examples of stress that many people have gone through at some point.

Healthy Coping Mechanisms

A good coping mechanism is a healthy way to make you feel better when you're stressed. There are a lot of different ones you can try. Some help you change the way you feel when you're stressed. Some examples are **meditation**, exercise, listening to music, writing in a journal, or doing a fun activity.

Other coping mechanisms help you fix a problem that's making you stressed. For example, if you have a lot of chores to do and you don't know how to start, making a to-do list might help. Other examples of this kind of coping mechanism are asking for help, taking a break, and logging off the internet.

Facing the Facts

Between 200 million and 500 million people around the world use meditation as a coping mechanism.

Doing something creative, dancing for fun, and watching a favorite TV show are all things someone might do to cope with stress. Not everyone will like every coping mechanism. Try different ones, and see what works for you!

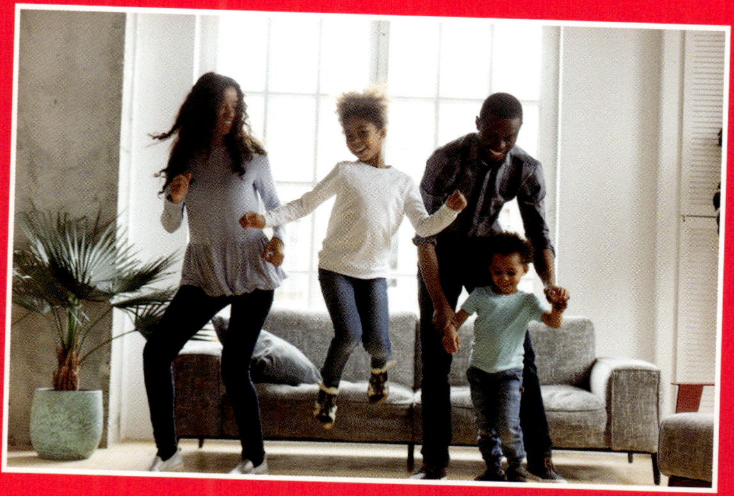

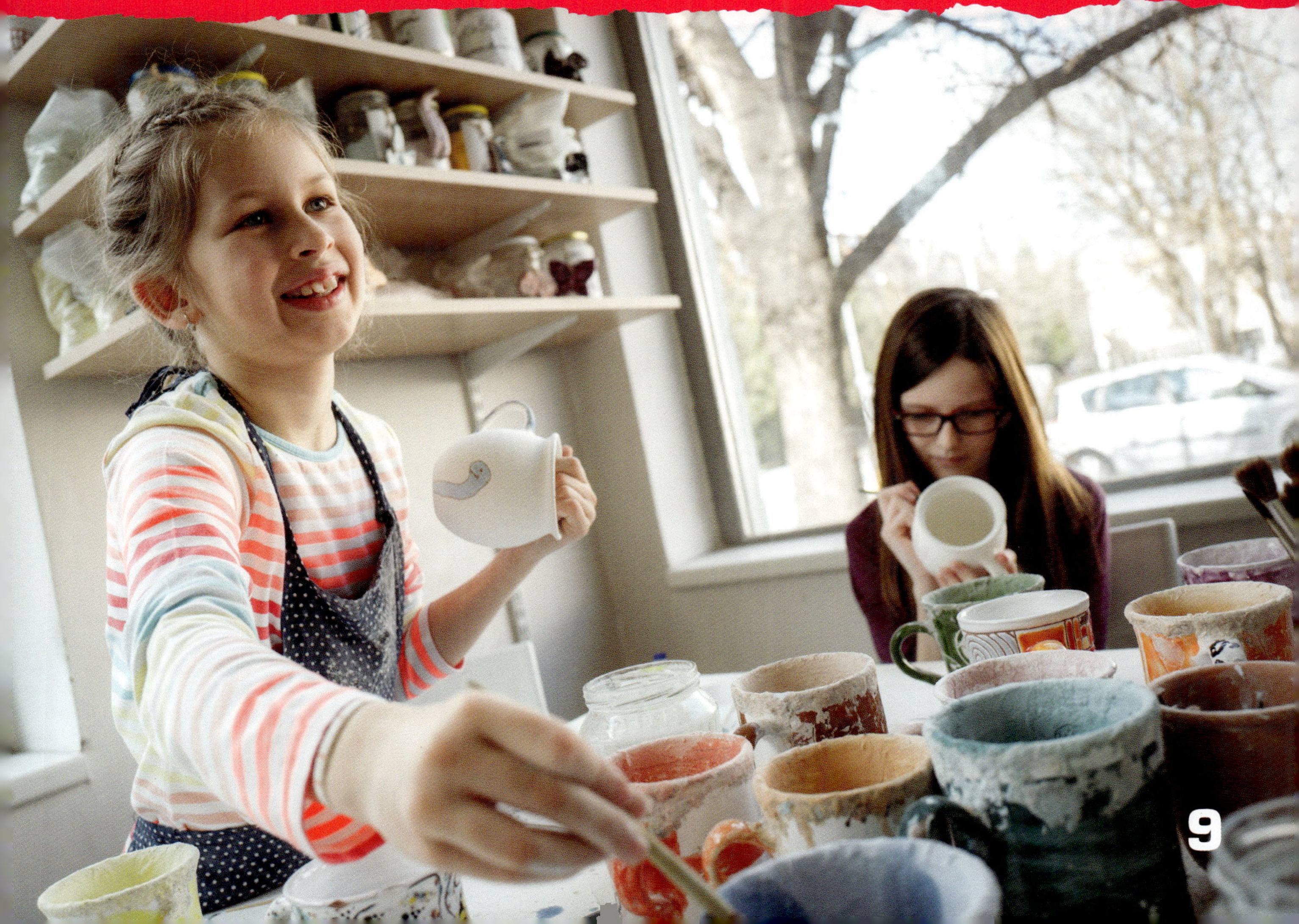

Unhealthy Coping Mechanisms

Poor coping mechanisms often feel good in the moment, but over time, they make your mental health worse. Often, they make your physical health worse too. One unhealthy coping mechanism a lot of people use is eating too much or too little. Others are using drugs or drinking. These coping mechanisms cause more problems than they fix.

Sometimes even a healthy coping mechanism can become unhealthy. For example, taking a break from homework to watch a video online can be a good way to make yourself feel less stressed. However, watching videos all night instead of doing any homework will just make you more stressed later.

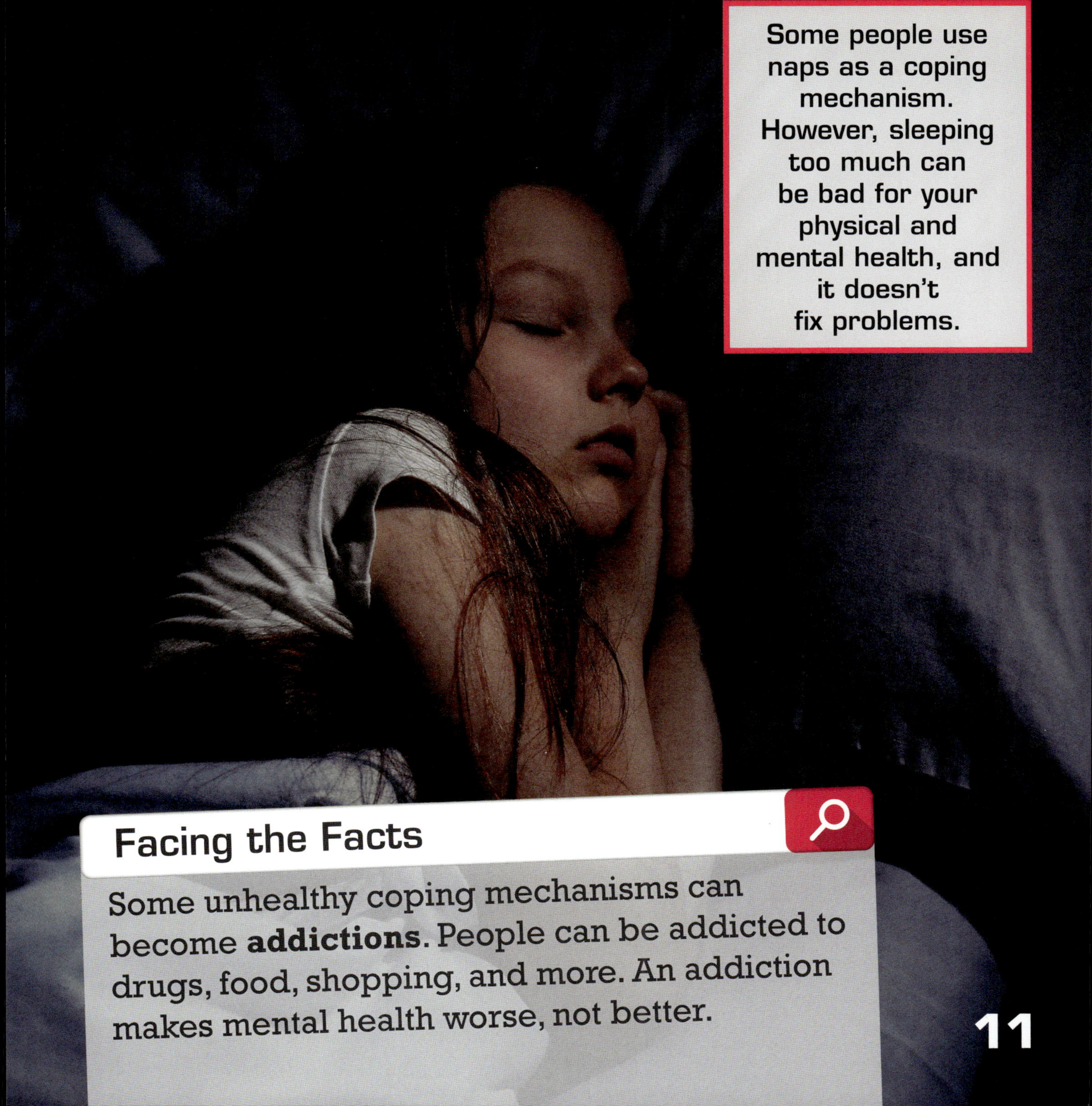

Some people use naps as a coping mechanism. However, sleeping too much can be bad for your physical and mental health, and it doesn't fix problems.

Facing the Facts

Some unhealthy coping mechanisms can become **addictions**. People can be addicted to drugs, food, shopping, and more. An addiction makes mental health worse, not better.

Setting Boundaries

Some healthy coping mechanisms might not feel good at first. One example is setting boundaries. These are rules you make for how other people can treat you. For example, if you have a friend who makes fun of you a lot in ways that upset you, you can set a boundary by telling them you won't spend time with them anymore if they keep doing it.

Setting a boundary can be stressful at first, so a lot of people avoid doing it. Some people get upset when other people set boundaries, but this doesn't mean boundaries are bad! Over time, setting boundaries leads to better mental health.

Facing the Facts

Setting boundaries is part of self-care, or things you do to take care of your health. Experts say one in three people feel guilty for taking time for themselves, but everyone needs to relax and take part in self-care!

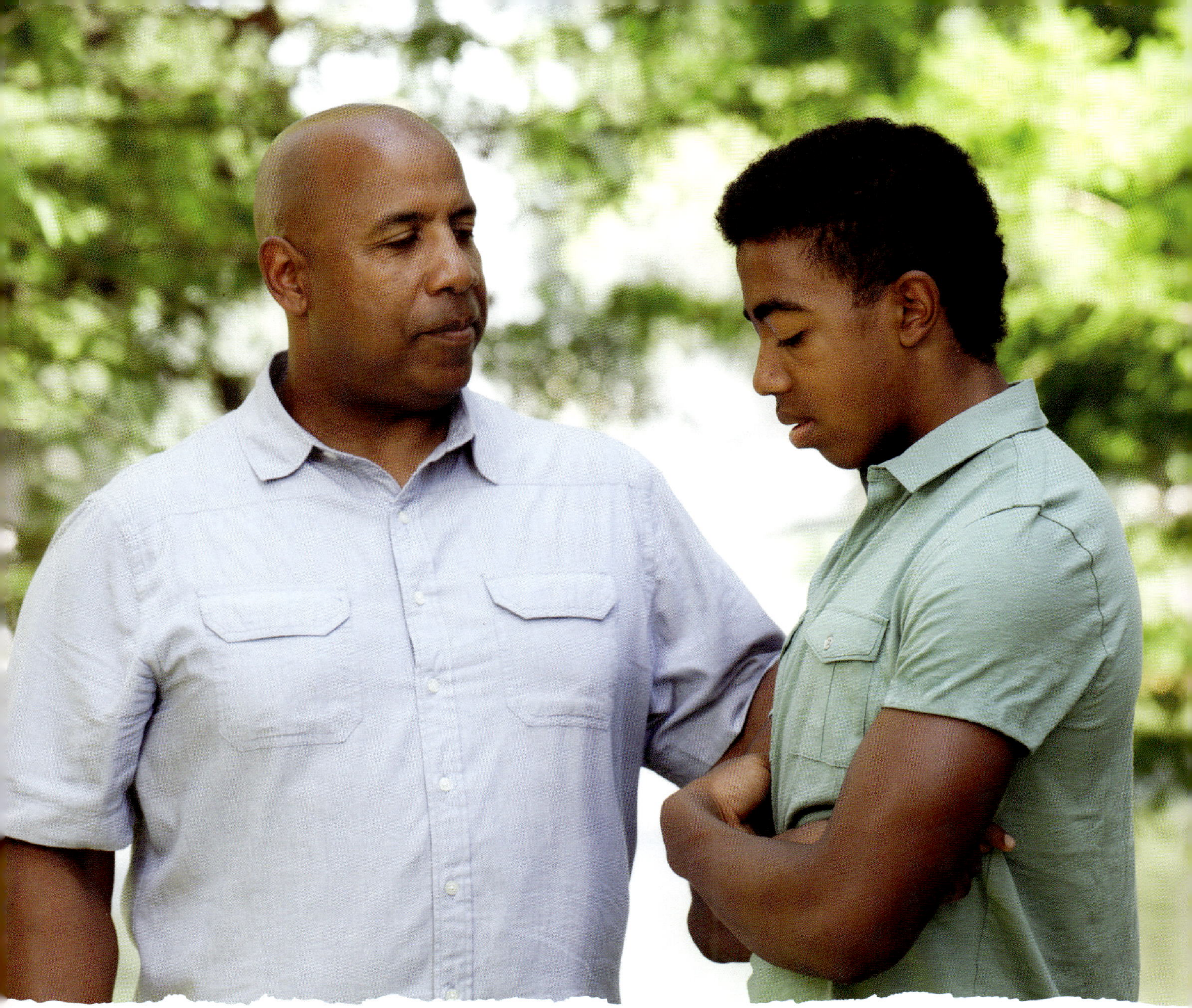

If setting boundaries seems scary or uncomfortable to you, talk to a trusted adult. They can help you find the right words to say and actions to take.

More Than Stress

Some people have poor mental health because they have a mental illness, or disorder. This is more than just stress. Experts aren't exactly sure what causes mental illnesses, but most think it has to do with a **chemical imbalance** in the brain.

Two of the most common mental illnesses are depression and anxiety. Depression makes people very sad, and anxiety makes them very nervous. Often, it seems like there's no reason for them to have these feelings. This makes it hard for a lot of people to understand someone else's mental illness.

Facing the Facts

About half of all people who have depression also have anxiety.

We all feel sad or nervous sometimes, but those feelings are only symptoms of a mental disorder if they go on for two or more weeks.

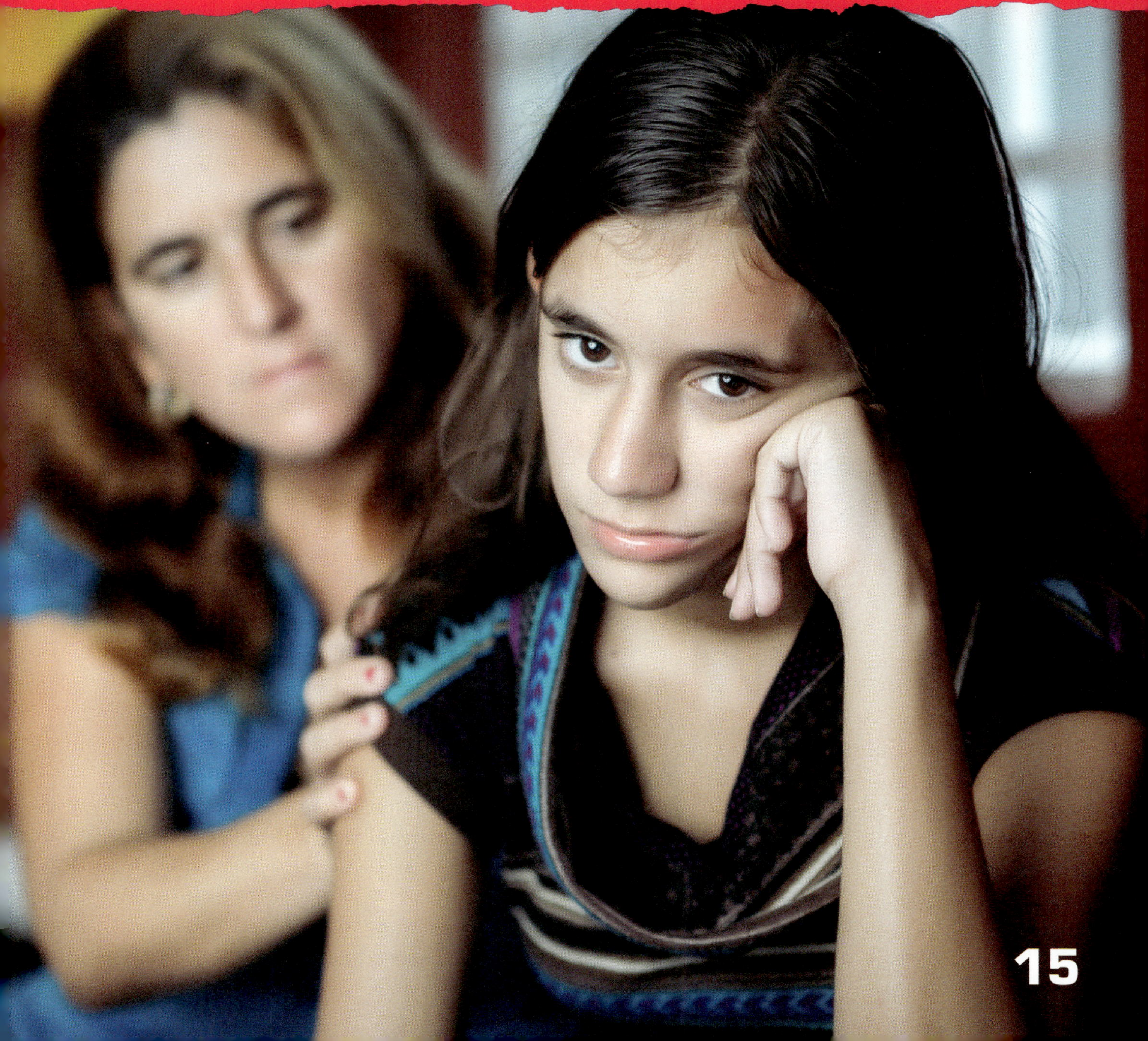

Dealing with Mental Illness

Because mental illnesses are different than stress, the ways people cope with them are also different. Meditation and exercise can help, but they can't completely cure a mental illness. Most people need a **therapist** to help them figure out what coping mechanisms will help them.

Some people also need to take medicine to treat their chemical imbalance. This is like taking medicine to treat a heart problem. Mental illnesses might seem confusing or scary, but they're just like physical illnesses. A person with a mental illness often doesn't look sick, but their illness is real.

Facing the Facts

There are more than 200 different mental disorders. People can have more than one.

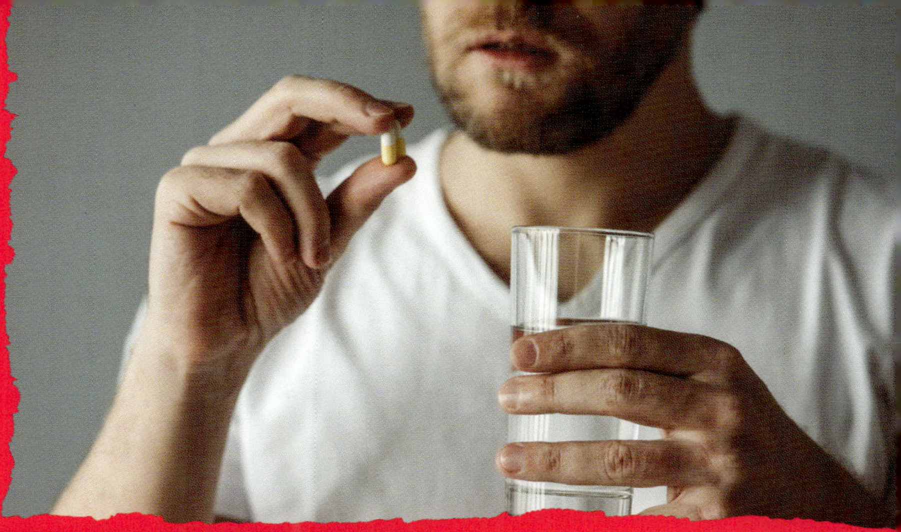

Talking to a therapist and taking medicine are two ways people can treat their mental illness. Many people do both.

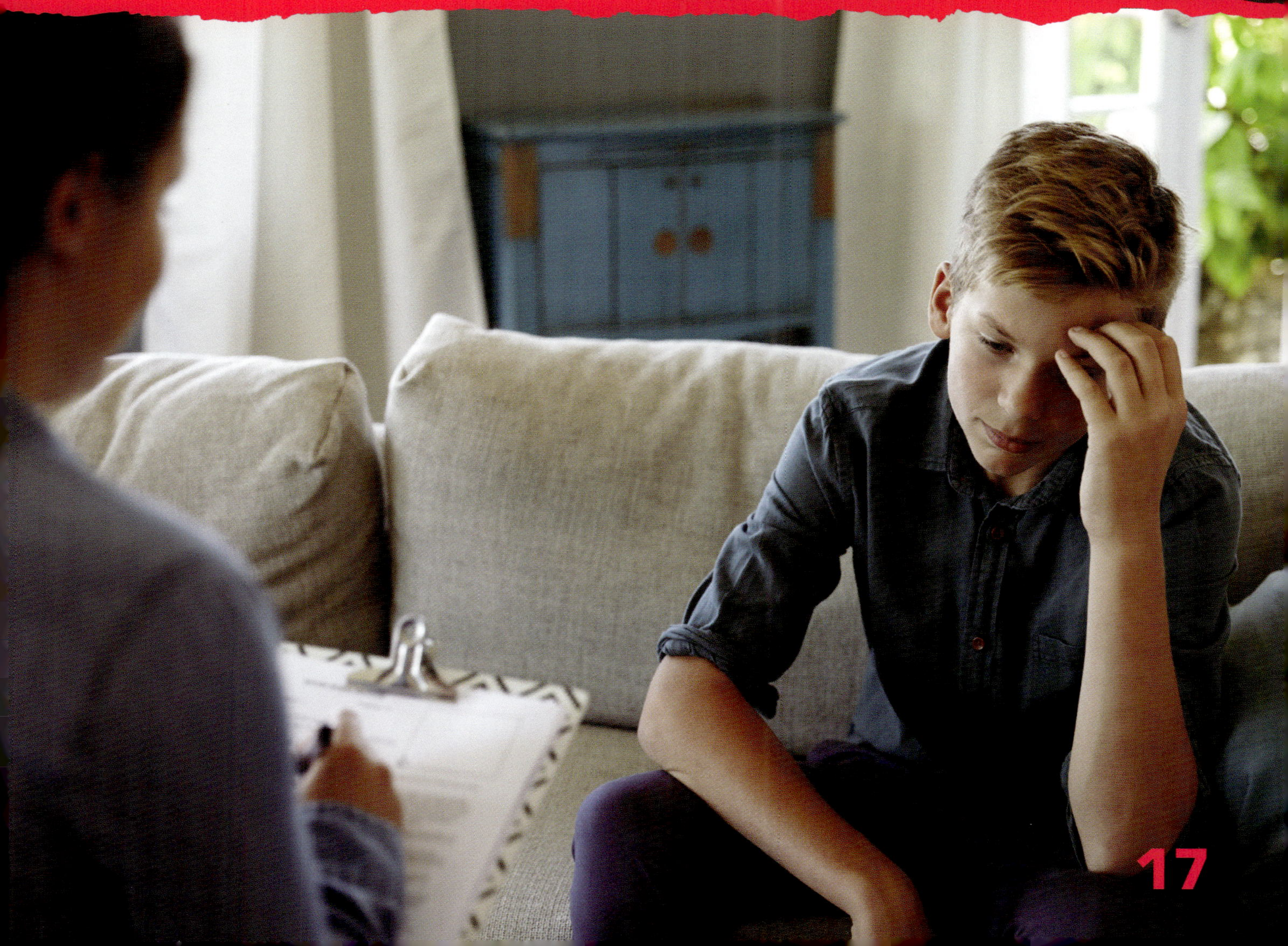

Symptoms of Poor Mental Health

Symptoms of poor mental health can be different for everyone. People who have a mental illness often have symptoms that are different or more **severe** than people who are just stressed. However, sometimes it can be hard to tell exactly why we don't feel good.

If you have symptoms of poor mental health, talk to a trusted adult about how you're feeling. They may be able to help you figure out what you can do to make your mental health better. There's nothing wrong with asking for help!

Facing the Facts

About 17 million young people in the United States have a mental health disorder. Half of them show symptoms before age 14.

Symptoms of POOR MENTAL HEALTH

- eating too much or too little
- sleeping too much or too little
- loss of interest in things you normally enjoy
- having more fights with friends and family
- feeling like nothing matters
- thinking of hurting yourself or someone else
- problems getting important chores done

If you have any of these symptoms, talk to someone about them. Everyone needs some help once in a while!

Taking Charge

Whether you're stressed or have a mental illness, there are things you can do to take charge of your mental health. If you think talking to a therapist would help you, ask your parent or guardian to help you find one. If you feel very stressed, try different healthy coping mechanisms until you find a few that work for you.

If you know someone who has a mental illness or is dealing with more stress than usual, try to be understanding. Ask them what you can do to help them. Remember that it's not their fault they feel this way. You can often be helpful just by listening to them.

Facing the Facts

Mental illness can affect anyone—even famous people. Dwayne "The Rock" Johnson, who was the voice of Maui in *Moana*, and singer Selena Gomez have struggled with depression.

WHAT CAN YOU DO?

Learn more about mental illness.

Listen respectfully when someone talks about their mental illness.

Pay attention to what makes you stressed so you can figure out how to cope.

Set mental health goals for yourself, such as setting aside time each day for self-care.

Set boundaries, and respect the boundaries other people set.

Take care of your physical health.

Use healthy coping mechanisms.

There are a lot of things you can do to take care of your mental health and be a good friend to someone who's having mental health problems.

GLOSSARY

addiction: A strong and harmful need to regularly have something or do something.

affect: To produce an effect on something.

chemical imbalance: Having too much or too little of the substances that control the way the brain works.

disorder: A physical or mental condition that is not normal or healthy.

expert: A person who has a special skill or knowledge.

meditation: Spending time in quiet thought, often paired with deep, slow breaths.

physical: Relating to the body.

severe: Very bad, serious, or unpleasant; causing a lot of pain or suffering.

stress: A state of strong feelings of worry.

therapist: A person who helps people deal with mental or emotional problems by talking about those problems.

FOR MORE INFORMATION

WEBSITES

BrainPOP: Mental Health

www.brainpop.com/health/mentalhealth

This section of the BrainPOP website includes information and activities about various aspects of mental health.

Gizmo's Pawesome Guide to Mental Health

www.preventsuicidect.org/wp-content/uploads/2012/08/GizmoPawesome.pdf

In this PDF e-book, Gizmo the therapy dog and his friends explain mental health. The book features a page for making a personal mental health plan.

BOOKS

Allen, Vanessa Green, and Sarah Rebar. *Me and My Feelings: A Kids' Guide to Understanding and Expressing Themselves*. Emeryville, CA: Rockridge Press, 2019.

Claybourne, Anna. *Self-Esteem and Mental Health*. London, UK: Franklin Watts, 2017.

Maddox, Lucy. *What Is Mental Health? And Other Big Questions*. London, UK: Wayland, 2020.

Publisher's note to educators and parents: Our editors have carefully reviewed these websites to ensure that they are suitable for students. Many websites change frequently, however, and we cannot guarantee that a site's future contents will continue to meet our high standards of quality and educational value. Be advised that students should be closely supervised whenever they access the Internet.

INDEX